PATRINA

THE SEXY BODY BLUEPRINT

SUNSHINE REIGN PUBLISHING

The Sexy Body Blueprint by Patrina Mosca

www.becommittedwellness.com

ISBN: 978-0-692-14987-4

Published by Sunshine Reign Publishing

Sunshine Regin Publishing
Houston, TX
sharon@mcwritingservices.com

Book Project Management:
The Master Communicator's Writing Service • www.mcwritingservices.com

Cover and Interior Design: D.E. West / ZAQ Designs

Printed in the United States of America

SUNSHINE REIGN PUBLISHING

DEDICATION

I want to dedicate this book to all the women out there who may have lost their way because of a terrible relationship, addiction, rejection, abuse, abandonment, sickness, a loss, or whatever has gotten you off course. Trust me you will be made whole. I found my Light in Jesus. He gave me the gift of fitness and I want to share the gift that He gave to me with you!

Ladies...push through, Light and Joy is on the other side!

#love

Patrina

CONTENTS

FOREWORD

I met Patrina Mosca when I presented her many awards at a fitness competition. She has graced the competition stage many times; winning multiple metals as a fitness competitor and is always a graceful and sparkling power on stage. When you speak to her in person, she is always humble, gracious and eager to help others. In her free time she runs boot camps and teaches classes in efforts to help others lose weight and become healthier.

I did not know the deeper roots of Patrina's story until reading her book. Behind her glamorous appearance and impeccable physique is a story of struggle and climbing back to survival. Her book gives a frank look at how after the death of her children's father, her life turned to substance abuse and how finding God's love was her wakeup call to turn her life around. Not only did the substance abuse stop, she changed her eating and exercise habits as well. She did a complete turn to change her life and health. From there she has become a fitness competitor, trainer, found love again, and wrote this book with the intent of helping others that may be in a similar situation she was. She has been through it all and has a non-judgmental approach to help others to live a healthier happier life. This book has transformed and inspired me in so many ways and I guarantee it will do the same for you as well.

For those of you that have lost hope in any area of your life, are suffering from substance abuse, struggling with weight issues, or similar areas, you will find inspiration in this book. Patrina is a survivor and will help many others not just survive but thrive through her words and inspiration. Her book is a celebration of her triumph to a healthy lifestyle and will guide you to do the same.

Dr. Regina A. Bailey, MD, JD

ACKNOWLEDGEMENTS

Dear God, my Creator, thank you for placing this purpose and calling on my life! To my husband Fausto, who tirelessly cheers me on; you are my gift and my blessing for life. You show me a dimension of love only a spouse can — I never understood THAT type of love until you came into my life. Your support and encouragement — I do not take for granted. Thank you, to my Momma who has loved me in my rebellion, when I was so difficult to love, you were there. Thank you for just being the beautiful and wise woman of God you are. To my children, who tell me, "Momma you can do anything." I believe them, and it is those words that propel me to accomplish my goals. To V. Essa Dodd, my most loving sister — you are my flower, encourager and the one who keeps me grounded.

I must thank my brother Cordale Baldwin who introduced me to the world of bodybuilding. He is my mentor, coach, and go to for all things fitness!!! The Lord told Cordale I would be a trainer first. Ha, ha!

...and to my lil Sister Crystal Lauderdale, thanks for your encouragement and love. "The Heavens are Open and They Are Open Over Us."

To my Spiritual Leaders, Pastor Keion Henderson and First Lady Felicia Henderson at the Lighthouse Church in Houston, thank you for mentoring me from afar. You have blessed my life in ways you will never know by providing me and others in the flock with the resources and contacts to help us accomplish our goals and be successful.

To my Coach Dawniel Winningham the business midwife! I wrote all this content three years ago. It's literally been sitting inside of a computer for 3 YEARS! When I met coach, she gave me the assignment and in one month this book has come to life. I can't thank you enough for kicking me in the pants and getting my behind to work. Coach, you are the absolute best and I can't wait to do more work!

To Ms. Sharon Jenkins my editor and literary guide throughout this entire process. Thank you for your gentleness, patience, and expertise. You made this journey so easy and fun!

I must acknowledge every client who has allowed me to be a part of their fitness journey. Past, present, and future clients, you have made me a better person and trainer. I appreciate you. Go for it!!!

INTRODUCTION

I am Patrina Mosca, wife, mother, lover of people and all things fitness. My children Jaylin, Mia, Jamila, Laura, and Allegra are my greatest contributions to this world. I am a native Houstonian and member of the Lighthouse Church under the leadership of Pastor Keion Henderson and First Lady Felicia Henderson. I love my church family! I love serving the elderly and those in need.

My husband, Fausto and I met right here in Houston. Running brought us together and our common passion is fitness. We train, meal prep, and run races together. Fausto is Italian, which makes our relationship so fun and unique. We enjoy blending our cultures and traditions.

I am an avid runner, but my favorite workouts take place in the weight rooms! I love to lift. My body responds well to weightlifting. It's the foundation of my company's training methods. I am a figure competitor. Fitness and figure competition is a class of physique-exhibition events for women, and I have placed and

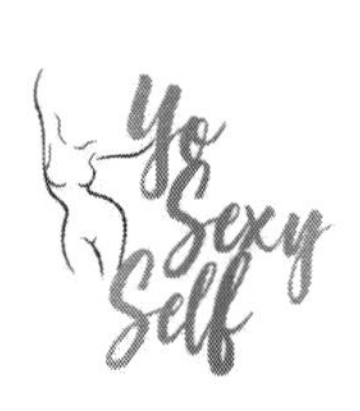

Fitness came to me during one of the lowest points of my life.

won in the NSL (Nspire Sports League) and Musclemannia natural leagues. I enjoy the competition process and the overall experience. I am a certified fitness trainer, nutritionist, and licensed massage therapist.

Fitness came to me during one of the lowest points of my life. It happened in two very distinct phases. February 25, 2007, Jamila and Laura's father passed away on Laura's 4th birthday. We were to have her party at his home and I found him there dead. He went to sleep and never woke up. I was shocked, upset, and hurt. Honestly, he helped me a lot with the kids and I thought to myself, "How in the world will I care for these kids 100% without his help?" I didn't want to be the sole provider because I wanted some freedom. I didn't want to be a full-time mother — I wanted to do it part-time. I was thinking about myself, not about what happened and the hurt and pain my children were feeling. I was selfish and delusional.

So I became a "functioning" alcoholic and drug user. I got my kids to and from school but had rum for breakfast. I paid our bills and made sure my children had what they needed but was not present mentally or emotionally. I went through the motions of life. Rum turned into weed — weed turned into ecstasy — ecstasy turned into cocaine and I turned into a hot mess.

I began to drink and smoke in front of my kids and I didn't care about the consequences. I would get angry if anyone confronted me about it. Through a series of events I came back to my senses like the Prodigal Son in Luke 15.

My girls has a godmother who would spend time with them on weekends. She taught children's church at Wheeler Ave Church here in Houston. She had the girls ask me to meet her at Wheeler to pick them up. I must be honest – I didn't want to step one foot inside of a church. I thought to myself, I am living so recklessly — I know God is mad at me and doesn't want me in His house like this. I kept telling myself I needed to clean up before I went back to church. I thought going to church in my present state was disrespectful. I didn't want to disrespect His house with my dirty presence. Those thoughts kept me away from church. I felt shame, nasty, and pitied myself, but this time I had to go. There was no way around it. The night before I had been partying, getting high, and was up all night. I vividly remember what I was wearing, a black flowered skirt and red blouse with strappy heel sandals. It was a hot morning and I was still high, but I remember Pastor Crosby preaching to the graduates. His sermon kept my attention. He talked about your inner circle and being on guard about the company you keep. I sat there – Honestly, I did not feel uncomfortable. My girls were not there – they were in children's church with their godmother. Right there while sitting in the pew Pastor's sermon was ending, and the Holy Spirit let loose. When He let loose – I stood up and began to shout, cry, run, and sweat. I jumped up and instantly I was sober. An older lady held me kissed me, and she told me I was going to be alright. I ran with such an intensity the shoes I had on broke. The heels, straps, everything – completely broke! That lady said something to me I will never forget, "Baby, God is going to bless you with so many pairs of new shoes now – your life will never be the same." Her smile comforted me. She hugged me and I truly felt welcomed into my new church family. I did not feel judged at all. I gathered my girls and talked to their godmother, she was happy because she was well aware of the train wreck I was. She was happy the girls were finally going to get a mother who would be present in their lives. I walked to my car knowing in my heart and soul that my life would never be the same. I had no idea what would happen next—what I did know was after that encounter with the Holy Spirit I couldn't go back, I must keep looking forward. I had to repent to my children. I asked my kids for forgiveness for not being a good mother to them. I talked privately to my eldest as I knew he understood the most. I forgave myself and I changed my circle IMMEDIATELY. No more partying friends – period! God had most of them vanish. So yes, I believe God looked down from

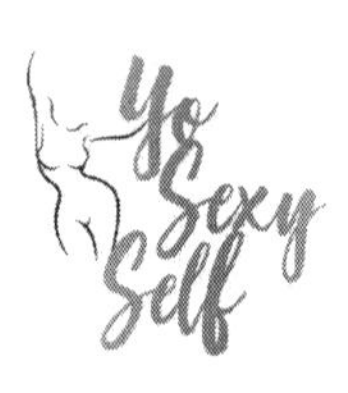

I knew then
I could no longer
live recklessly.

heaven on me and said, "Daughter that's enough!" He rescued me because I could not stop and He placed new desires in my heart. One was the desire to take care of myself through fitness — I received a visitation from the Holy Spirit, He came to me and pulled me up. I honestly could not have done it — He did.

I knew then I could no longer live recklessly. I tell people, I lived without a conscience. Well, the Holy Spirit placed a conscience and awareness inside of me I did not previously have. I got rid of all of my drugs and drug paraphernalia and I began to do what I thought good mothers do.

No more fast food all the time, I was cooking family dinners. I would take them on outings and attend church with them. We did homework together, I listened to them, showered them with love, and totally denied my previous addiction any control over my life.

I joined a gym to give me something to do with the time I usually partied. So I went from dropping my kids off at school and going to the liquor store to going to the gym. The gym was new and honestly not very exciting at first, but I was determined to like it. I hired a trainer there to help me get my feet wet. The members there were very nice and it felt like a community. I made new friends — and although I wasn't in good shape I continued to show up. I felt better over time. Did I think about getting high or drinking? Of course, I did, but whenever I thought about reverting back to my old ways — I thought about my children and I refused to disappoint them.

There was a park near my children's school. When the weather was good I would go for walks there. I thought to myself — I passed this park a million times before and never even thought once about walking the trails. It's funny how something you've always needed in your life to help you is right in front of you. I initially started off walking and then one day I jogged because I saw some other people jogging. (I am a competitor by nature.)

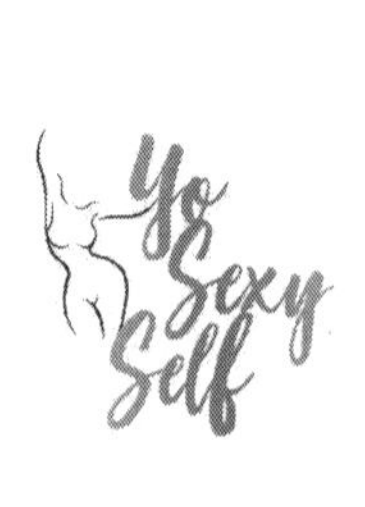

I have been in your shoes — I know how hard it is to decide to make a complete 180-degree turn in one's life...

I started out doing a quarter mile. Over time it increased to a mile and then a few more. My sense of accomplishment kept me going. People around me started to recognize my progress and began to encourage me. In addition to their support, I was being led by the Holy Spirit to do these things.

I began to go to different grocery stores to be introduced to new foods. I knew soul food, but I was curious about other foods. So I ventured out of my neighborhood to other communities to see what they ate. I wanted to know how to prepare healthier foods for my family. I exposed myself to new things and ideas.

And this is where I really started my change.

My story may not sound exactly like yours, but what we both can relate to is a struggle and I know it's difficult to just start. I knew all that time while I was in darkness I wasn't being kind to my body but I didn't know how to stop. My passion for this comes from the struggle I had. Depression, grief, and feeling lonely pushed me in the wrong direction and I started making wrong choices.

I have been in your shoes — I know how hard it is to decide to make a complete 180-degree turn in one's life — and to be honest my change is still happening. This is a daily walk — I put one foot in front of the other focusing only on today. I try not to overthink it or look too far ahead because I don't want to get too overconfident or tripped up. So I pray daily for a renewal of my mind and ask for the new grace and mercy which my Bible tells me God gives us every morning.

How do you eat an elephant? One bite at a time. That is what I do, take small bites of life and try not to digest huge chunks. I could choke or throw up. This book is your small bite. I want to give you insight, guidance, and information to consider when beginning your journey. These are the tools I would have liked to have known early on as I started getting healthy. They are my contribution to your establishing a great foundation for a successful lifestyle change. I want to mentor you through this process and save you time and money! Let's get through this phase then move on to the next.

The word of God says — *Time and chance happen to them all.* (Ecclesiastes 9:11) Well, this is your time and chance. Make the change!

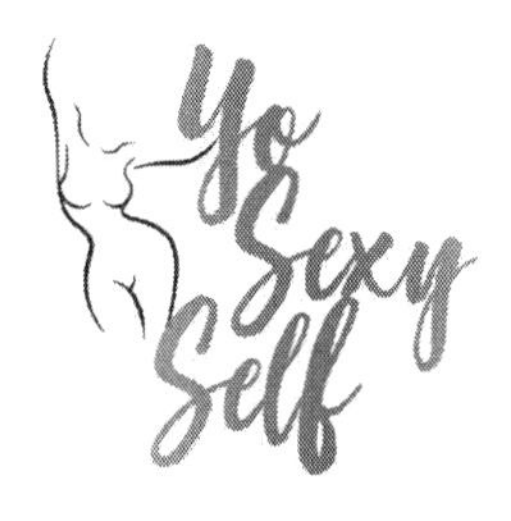

MAKING the COMMITMENT

Section One

ESTABLISHING YOUR WHY, WHAT, HOW, and WHO

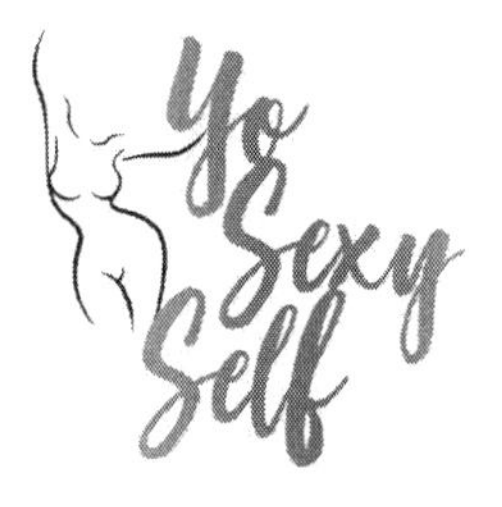

WHY?

Why now? What is your motivation for this journey? What has been one moment or event that happened in your life – that made you go, "Okay it's time!"

For me it happened one day during the winter, I looked at myself in a full-length mirror, my husband walked in and I felt embarrassed. I did not want him to see me naked. Up until that moment we had always been free around one another naked but, – that day I saw myself in the daylight looking like an out of shape woman who'd been neglecting herself. I covered up like Adam and Eve did when they sinned in the garden of Eden. I felt ashamed of how I, Me, Patrina let my body go. I did not feel sexy or desirable. As I looked at my out of shape body, I thought, "I wouldn't want to make love to this body, then why would he?" I knew – I had to do something to change my physical appearance. That day I made my mind up to #besexy for my husband. Yeah it was important to me, but to be honest I wanted to be desirable to him.

COMPETITION

Competitions are a great place to start. You have a date which will keep you accountable. If you register for a 5k, 10k, or half-marathon, you will be more likely to commit to your running schedule – because the dollars have been spent. Also knowing others are somewhere doing the same kind of preparation to perform the same task will push you!

Races and fitness competitions provide great communities where you gain friends who are like minded. Trade training strategies, and/or discuss opportunities.

Types of Competition

- 5K
- 10K
- Half or Full Marathon Ironman
- Strongman
- Personal Best CrossFit
- Pageant
- Dance
- Fitness Competition
- Weight Loss Competitions

SOCIAL

Now this is a big one! Oh, I'm getting married next year I need to lose weight. I love it! I did the same thing years ago.

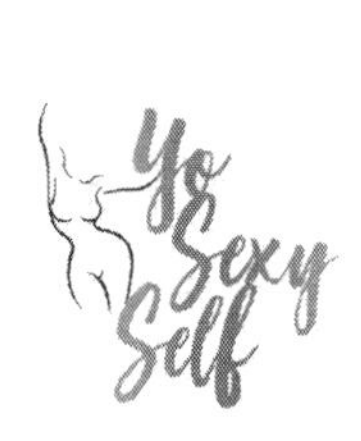

Races and fitness competitions provide great communities where you gain friends who are like minded.

It's okay. That can be a reason to start, but the "gotcha" is you don't get to stop after the wedding. You must continue. Anniversaries are another great reason to get rid of your excess weight. As I write this book my husband and I are getting ready to celebrate our 8th year of marriage. We are going to a beach somewhere in Mexico and you can best believe I have been doing extra to look cute in my swimsuit. So having an anniversary coming up is a great reason to get started but again you must keep up the work after the celebration. I never stopped, I just turned it up from 7 to 10!

Class reunions are another good reason. I am 40 now, and to be honest my body is in better shape than when I was in high school. I don't have youth – but I am physically stronger, and my endurance levels are high. I could not run 13 miles in high school, but I can now. So it's important to know that you may not be able to be that size 5 that you were in the 11th grade. But you can redefine the body you presently have to a more healthier state. Most of us have children, jobs, spouse – we didn't have any of that in high school or college so – let's be real. Start because of your class reunion and REMEMBER keep up the work after the reunion!

Types of Social Occasions which Act as Motivators

- Class Reunion
- Wedding
- Anniversary
- Birthdays

MEDICAL DESPERATION OR INSPIRATION?

These two motivators typically drive individuals to make lifestyle changes. They either get inspired by someone else's story or journey. For example, they may see a loved one or co-worker who followed the process and it changed their lives. So they may decide, "Hey I will give this a try." Simply because they witnessed

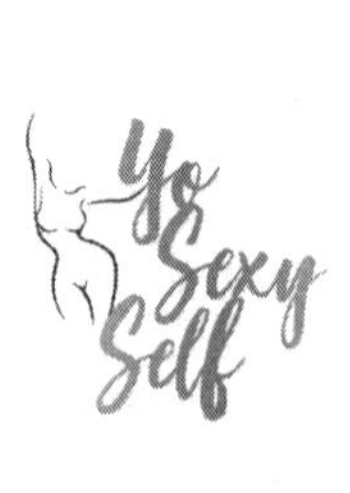

So it's important to know that you may not be able to be that size 5 that you were in the 11th grade. But you can redefine the body you presently have to a more healthier state.

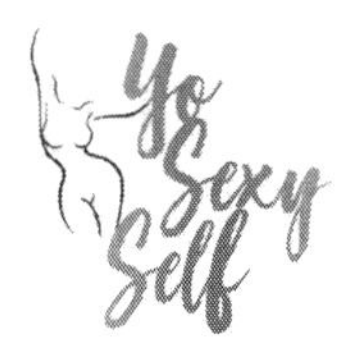

> You become desperate because you want to live.

it firsthand. This gives them the proof and hope they need to attempt to lead a healthier lifestyle.

Another cause for concern comes when you get bad news from your physician. That news may sound something like what Whoopi Goldberg told Demi Moore in Ghost, "YOU IN DANGER GIRL!" Suddenly you become scared and feel pushed to make a drastic change. It's life or death? You become desperate because you want to live. You sometimes just want to live a good quality life. So you finally make up your mind and do what you should have been doing years ago. You chose the healthy road.

Don't decide because of desperation – be inspired. Get the inspiration from someone or even find it within yourself!

Types of Medical Desperation

- Desire to Conceive,
- Improve Blood Pressure
- Joint Mobility
- Diabetes
- Cholesterol
- Mental Clarity
- Self Esteem

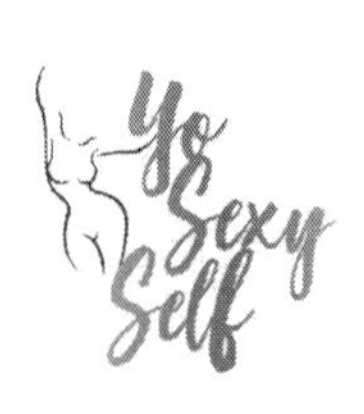

The truth is many jobs will require you to be in shape and have your physical appearance intact.

OCCUPATION

The truth is many jobs will require you to be in shape and have your physical appearance intact. It's the presentation that is important. Example, a real estate agent must show homes and convince people to buy. I recently had one call me because the task of showing homes in hot Houston was wearing on them and they wanted to build stamina and endurance to be able to work a full day with more ease.

I even had a disc jockey hire me because he wanted to improve his image to get more jobs. His image was his body. Building some muscle, leaning down, and looking more fit contributed to his success.

When going on an interview, employers are looking to see what kind of shape you're in. They don't want to hire someone who may "look" like they could be calling in sick a lot or may not be physically fit to perform their job duties.

Occupational Goals

- Apply for Military
- Interview for a Job
- Healthy Job Travel

Remember your need to be healthy should be your on-going motivation. The weight loss or healthier body will be the result of your why. Wanting to lose weight alone won't be enough to sustain your results. It will be temporary. Allow the weight loss be your outcome – not the main target!

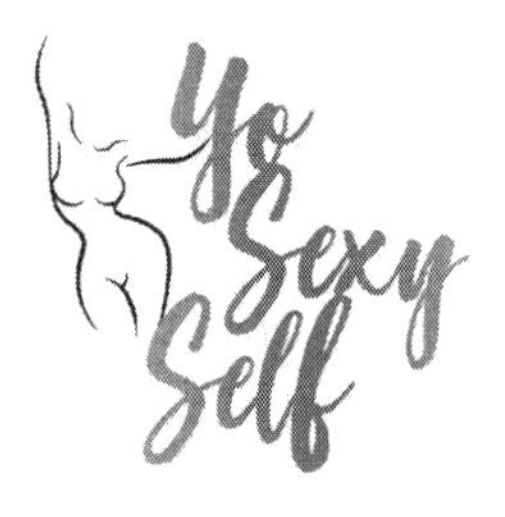

WHAT?

THE CAUSE

There is an old saying, "We are what we eat," but there are both internal and external sources which provoke us to eat in an unhealthy manner. Once you identify the cause or trigger, you can also conquer it and be well on your way to living the healthy lifestyle you desire.

Genetics is the study of heredity and the variation of inherited characteristics. Simply speaking, genetics say what you can be but not what you will be when it comes to maintaining your weight and weight loss. Don't allow your genetics to be an excuse for being overweight. My mother, grandmother, and great-grandmother were all obese. Although I have their genetics, I decided to be proactive and not allow this to be my reason for being out of shape. With the right blueprint you can combat genetics and get the body you want.

Bad or unhealthy relationships can definitely play a part in weight gain and become an obstacle to weight-loss. I have seen it firsthand. For example, a lady decides after years of marriage she wants to improve her physical appearance. She wants to lose some weight, highlight her hair, and spend time on self-care. Her spouse all of a sudden feels threatened and immediately tries to sabotage her efforts. She leaves in the early morning to work out. Her husband and their small children are still asleep. He wakes up early to go to work, leaving the children at home, then calls to let her know the kids are alone and she needs to end her workout. Now he knew she scheduled that time to improve herself, but he wants to sabotage her efforts. The husband creates adverse environmental conditions to make it difficult for her to achieve her goals. (Relationships like this one are normally fractured.)

Also, some of your longtime friends will discover you want to make a change and get jealous or just not care you are deciding to do some new things for yourself.

You could hear, "Oh now you're too good to go to happy hour with us?"

"Seems like all you want to do is hang out in the gym and workout?" Don't be discouraged, it's okay your goals are not their goals. Friends should support other friends doing positive things. I am not saying you should ditch your friends but be mindful and pay attention if the comments just don't stop. You will find new likeminded friends in your new gym.

The other bad relationship you must address is YOUR RELATIONSHIP with food. Sorry (not really), I dislike the term comfort food. Food is not supposed to comfort you. We have all used it to make us feel better about life, but that's not the purpose of food. It is to nourish you. The Be Committed Wellness philosophy is to teach our clients to eat for their goals. Learn the benefits of what to eat, when to eat it, and how much.

Don't abuse food. YES!!!! you can abuse food just like drugs or alcohol because the abuse of it can make you sick!

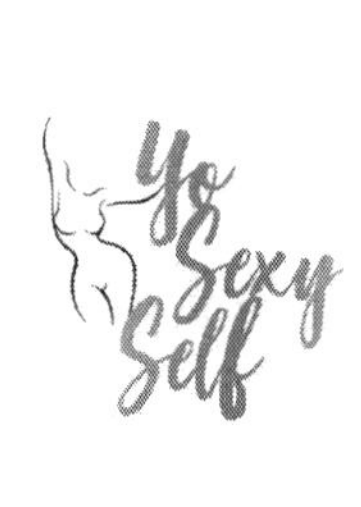

Bad or unhealthy relationships can definitely play a part in weight gain and become an obstacle to weight-loss.

Food is not a lover. You would be surprised how many people who get into a lonely place and then reach over for a bowl of ice cream to comfort and console them. It's unhealthy.

Trauma is another trigger. I binge watch the show My 600lb Life. It is very interesting to see a person's journey of how they ate themselves to 600 plus pounds and if they make up their minds most of them actually lose a lot of weight.

One common issue with both men and women on the show

is some childhood trauma and sexual abuse. Most say they ate to create a barrier between them and society so they wouldn't be attractive and no one would abuse them again. It's a sad reality. If you have been abused – seek professional help to uncover the layers to put you on a path of emotional healing. Start there, that help coupled with this book and my other resource you can lose the weight, but you must address the trauma which took place.

Your lifestyle could also be a contributor to your weight gain. Living for the weekend, partying, being sedentary, and constantly eating at restaurants packs on the pounds over time. That changes today!

This is a cause is near and dear to my heart because one of the reasons I ended up overweight in the first place is, I centered every date and celebration around food. I felt like I had to until a light bulb went off in my head. My husband and I love running. So I decided to plan a date at Memorial Park where we would have a

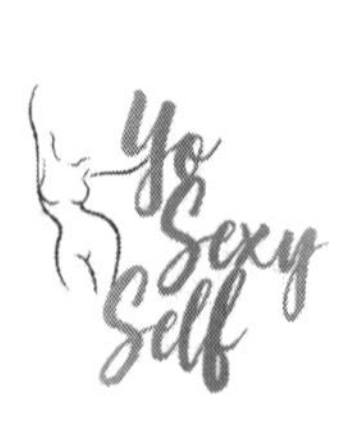

You must exercise discipline in order to have success for this journey.

nice run then go to a nearby Whole Foods and enjoy a healthy post run meal. He loved it and so did I. After exercise, your endorphins are high and your body is feeling good. It heightens the "loving" feeling you have for each other. So I changed the setting of our dates. We didn't stop having them we simply changed the location.

A lack of discipline could also be a major contributor to your unhealthy lifestyle. Let's be honest I think we all STRUGGLE with self-discipline because what's better than an Oreo, I will tell you a DOUBLE STUFFED OREO. I loved double stuffed Oreos, but they are not good for me. I am a sugar addict. I know it. I have come to grips with it. My way to deal with it is to take breaks by going cold turkey. I decided to say to myself in October, "Patrina that's enough. No more Oreos until your birthday." Then it truly is a treat and my anticipation grows as I get closer to the date.

Self-Control is a fruit of the Spirit. When I pray in the morning I ask God to please give me self-control over my body, finances, tongue, and my mind. I have to renew it every day. Because what I could resist yesterday maybe extra hard today.

You must exercise discipline in order to have success for this journey.

Identifying causes and triggers to your unhealthy lifestyle

- Genetics
- Bad Relationships
- Trauma

- Change in Career
- Lifestyle
- Being Undisciplined

MOTIVATION

What is your motivation? What will push you beyond your current norm to pursue a higher quality life? Weight loss should be a consequence of your goal, NOT the goal. Your reason for beginning this journey should be your own not someone else's. You have to do the work so there has to be a motivation and passion fueled by you. At the end of the day, people will have their opinions and that's fine, but this is your body and you only get one. Our life is not a dress rehearsal for another one. This is it.

Deciding to go on this journey just to get skinny is probably not the best approach. Get healthy, get strong, and fall in love with a new lifestyle. Thinking this way relieves the pressure. At my smallest I have not been "skinny" but I have been my strongest physically!

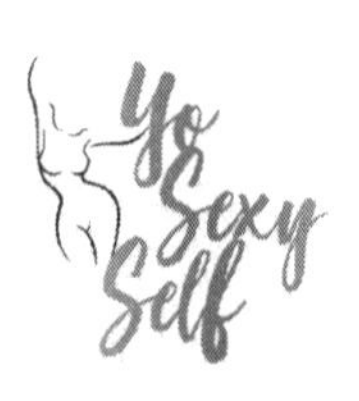

> Weight loss should be a consequence of your goal, NOT the goal.

Your plan should not be a one size fits all. My philosophy with my clients and myself when it comes to eating and training is; we train and eat for our goals. Some people are on plans which are not set for their goals. There's muscle building plans, weight loss plans, plans to build muscle while losing fat, and there are weight gain plans. What if you are not interested in anything regarding your weight but you want to increase your endurance and run a half marathon? That calls for an altogether different plan. See where I am going. If you want to build some muscle and lose fat you can't do a liquid diet – it won't get you the desired results.

It's important to be specific with your coach on what it is you are looking to achieve to get the proper blueprint for a successful execution. There are a plethora of diets online but those are more or less "examples." So stay away from cookie cutter diets and choose the ONE for you! Otherwise you may experience some serious frustration and waste valuable time doing the wrong thing which can cause discouragement. Get the right plan! Let's be fair you didn't gain 30lbs in a month so why expect to lose it in a month? Sometimes we have unrealistic expectations when trying to get fit. This process really isn't a process, but more like establishing new life habits you will continue to do so be patience please.

I am the mother of five and mothers can attest to this, it seems like children grow overnight – especially at the end of summer. They have slept in late and annihilated the refrigerator and pantry!

Then when it's time to buy clothes for school as the new year begins they have shot up 2 inches and their foot size has gone up drastically! You didn't see them grow, but they did. Nature nurtured them with food and lots of sleep and your children grew.

It's the same concept with weight loss, if you stick to the plan, be consistent and patient the weight WILL come off. Now if you stand in the mirror – you won't see yourself shrinking or melting but gradually as you get on the scale the number will go down. Your clothes will start to get loose. It will just happen.

Anything worth having will be a challenge. Know going in especially in the beginning this will not be easy. It's going to take you getting your mind right first. Once you make up in your mind that you are doing it – just jump! Jump in feet first into this new world, your new world knowing you have a goal to accomplish.

Our body will do what our minds tell it. I heard a saying, "If you say you can do it, you're right. If you say you can't do it, you're right." I don't know about you, but I want to be the one who said I can. If you are reading this book you have already decided you can do it. So do it.

Support is important and it helps fuel this goal. However if you just don't have it – it's not an excuse to fail. Seriously, I had to hold myself up many times when there was no one else there to prop me up. There is a verse in the Bible that says that David encouraged himself in the Lord. (1 Samuel 30:6) I think about

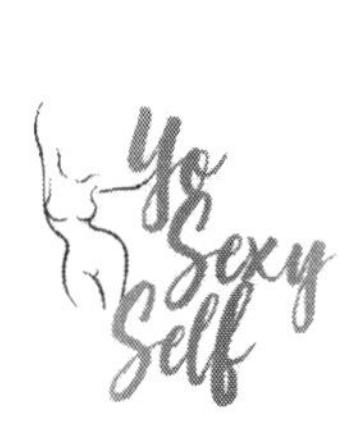

It's important to be specific with your coach on what it is you are looking to achieve to get the proper blueprint for a successful execution.

that when things become difficult and I call someone and they don't answer, I don't get upset. I encourage myself in the Lord.

Everyone won't understand what you're doing. This is new to you and to them. It's okay because this is your choice, you

made for yourself, a healthy and positive choice. Own it and do it with them or without them but you owe it to yourself.

OUTCOME GOALS

- This is a MARATHON not a sprint!
- Commit to your goal at least one calendar year!
- Statistics show two out of five individuals starting a "diet" quit in the first week!

One out of five last a month.[1]

The reasons "Why?"

- Wrong motivation
- Wrong plan
- Not seeing INSTANT results
- Not mentally prepared for the change
- No support

1. *"5 Reasons Most Diets Fail Within 7 Days,"* Health.com, accessed May 08, 2018, http://www.health.com/nutrition/5-reasons-most-diets-fail-within-7-days.

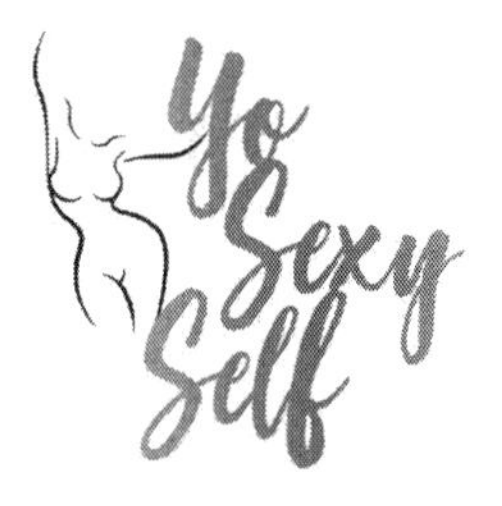

HOW?

How will you get this goal accomplished? The first thing I did was make up my mind. Then I reconciled in my mind I would have to invest time and money for this to happen for me. Patience is key. You didn't gain your weight in one month. It will take time to get the weight off. Some people have been gaining weight for years and will start a journey and think the weight will disappear in weeks. Come on now that is not reasonable.

You may ask, "How do I start?" First see a doctor before be-

Patience is key.
You didn't gain your weight in one month.
It will take time to get the weight off.

---

ginning any new weight-loss regime. Once you get clearance from your doctor, START!

Change your MIND! Again, change has to come mentally, then physically! Literally see yourself accomplishing this goal. Accept in your mind this WILL NOT be easy, but you WILL DO IT! Then make your mind up, NO MORE EXCUSES. Bombard your mind with information on healthy living, eating, exercise and positive thoughts about the new you.

As a nation, we underrate sleep. Your body needs sleep. It's essential to your body's recovery, mental health, and even your weight. When you sleep your body has a chance to regenerate dead cells, heal and repair. The National Sleep Foundation states that an adult person's body requires 7-9 hours of sleep per night.

The majority of people who are not living their healthiest lives experience two issues, 1. Lack of sleep and 2. Constipation (another chapter).

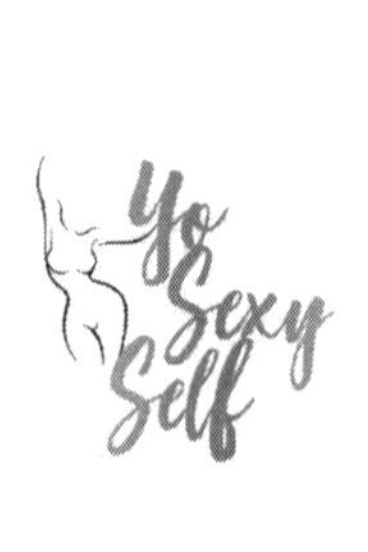

If you have a stressful career or life, have a scheduled time where you shut everything down and go to bed!

If you have a stressful career or life, have a scheduled time where you shut everything down and go to bed! Otherwise you will find yourself going on and on exhausting yourself – when the laundry or email could probably wait another 10 hours. You have to make getting enough sleep a priority. SLEEP will be essential to you achieving your goal.

I tell my clients all the time, if you don't power down, reset, and get adequate rest your body will SHUT DOWN. It's a matter of time. When they don't take the advice their immune system gets weak and here comes the colds, falling asleep at traffic lights, and their productivity and creativity decreases.

Get socially active! Create new goals, circles, and a new body will soon be yours. Know everyone will not understand, at first. You may lose some friends and gain new ones.

Also change your relationship with food. Be prepared to take your food with you. Learn how to co-exist with food.

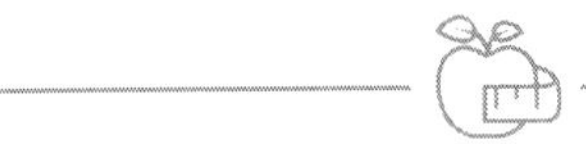

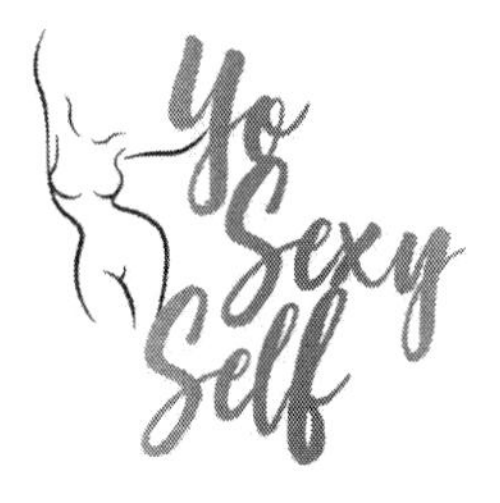

WHO?

Who will help you reach your goal(s)? I hired a professional trainer to help guide me through this journey. I had a gym membership but did not know how to properly work out. My trainer worked my body out according to my fitness goals. So I lost some weight BUT hit a plateau, so a nutritionist was necessary. Before hiring a professional trainer always schedule a consultation and assessment. This is a great opportunity to meet your prospective trainer to make sure your personalities match, scheduling matches your availability, and you also want to check credentials. This is the perfect time to get weighed, find out body fat percentages, and do initial fitness evaluation. This enables you to get a good picture of the start for your fitness journey.

THE BENEFITS OF A TRAINER

Having a trainer can be the difference between success and failure for your health. They hold you accountable – and will help you keep your body image in perspective. The next step would be

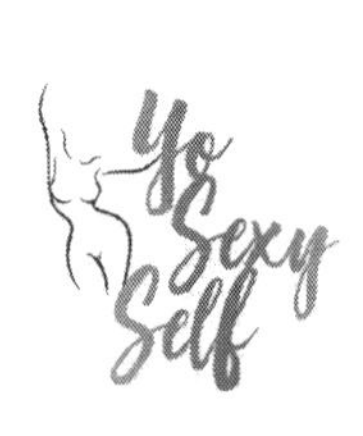

Before hiring a professional trainer always schedule a consultation and assessment.

to create custom workouts for your current fitness levels. Weight or Resistance training, conditioning, and endurance training are a few modalities we use at Be Committed Wellness. It provides the variety your body will need for muscle confusion to get maximize results! Trainers show you the correct form and how to perfectly perform an exercise and prevent injuries. They also help you break through a plateau and keep you motivated. A trainer can act as a counselor when you hit an obstacle and maximize your workout session. Trainers can also relate to your challenges and present you with right solutions because of their experience.

In training my motto is bend but don't break! You need to be challenged to get your body stronger but not injured. This constant challenging will keep the fat burning and the weight melting on!

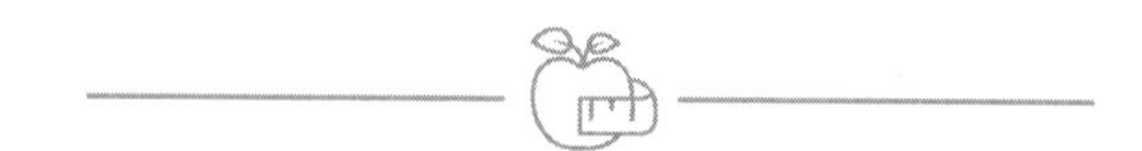

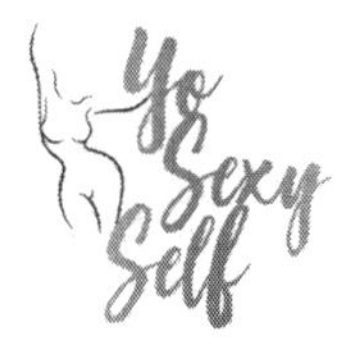

YOUR ADVOCATES DURING YOUR SEXY BODY JOURNEY

- GOD
- You
- Family
- Circle of Friends

This decision is yours. You are the one who will accomplish this goal. Some days you will have to motivate yourself. You are responsible for your journey. You can DO IT!

POTENTIAL MEMBERS OF YOUR ACCOUNTABILITY CIRCLE

- Workout partner
- Run Group / Team / Association
- Find someone who has reached your goal!
- Surround yourself with positive / uplifting individuals
- Embrace diversity

GOD IS YOUR #1 MOTIVATOR

- Find your STRENGTH in GOD!
- Chose a scripture to encourage yourself….
  REPEAT IT DAILY!
- Read your bible every day. Eat your daily bread!
- You cannot do this in the flesh, you need God.
- He is our STRENGTH.
- He cares for you and the matters of your heart.

SCRIPTURES THAT HELP ME GET THROUGH MY JOURNEY

When I first looked at my body and was truly dissatisfied and unhappy this verse always helped me to look beyond what I saw in the mirror.

Therefore, I urge you, brothers and sisters, in view of God's Mercy, to offer your bodies as a living sacrifice, holy and pleasing to God – this is your true and proper worship. - Romans 12:1

This verse helped me focus on my "why." My body is not my own but God's and I am to worship Him with it by treating it right. Taking good care of the temple He gave me is a spiritual mandate. I want to freely jump, run, and dance for Him. I want to be able to physically do worship in those ways. Being fit enables me to worship God in a way that brings glory to Him and pleases me.

Do you not know that your bodies are temples of the Holy Spirit, who is in you, whom you have received from God? You are not your own;... - 1 Cor 6:19

This scripture is one I pray every day! It is so important for me because it speaks to an issue that most of us suffer from, not only regarding wellness but also in other parts of our lives. Self-control is big for me, without it we all would be living in such excess that would be so unhealthy and unproductive. I pray this prayer daily because I don't always want to be kind to someone, but I must because my Father requires that of His children. So as I am to be kind, faithful, good, walk in peace: love, joy, and forbearance (restraint and tolerance). I must also exercise self-control. What has also helped me is thinking about it and telling myself, "Patrina exercise self-control." Sometimes I repeat it to myself several times so that it can get into my spirit.

But the fruit of the Spirit is love, joy, peace, forbearance, kindness, goodness, faithfulness, 23 gentleness and self-control. Against such things there is no law. - Galatian 5:22-23

This verse helps me when I am hungry, and I am not due for another meal for another hour or two. Hunger is real, but most time a glass of water or a verse like this one can help you overcome that sensation.

For our light affliction, which is but for a moment, worketh for us a far more exceeding an eternal weight of glory. - 2 Cor 4:17

Hunger is a light affliction and it flees. Keep your goal in mind and know that sometimes - NOT ALL of the time, you will feel some discomfort in this lifestyle change.

This is scripture is one of my favorites and very well known:

Jesus answered, "It is written: 'Man shall not live on bread alone, but on every word that comes from the mouth of God.'" - Mat 4:4

During fasting, or just when I pray over my food — I remind myself that this is just food. I need and want that word from God for my primary sustenance. Food is not a replacement.

Because you can eat what you want to eat, doesn't mean you should.

"Everything is permissible for me," but not everything is beneficial. - 1 Cor 6: 12

You can go out and eat this or that, or do this or that, but it doesn't mean that you should. This is where the self-control comes into play. I don't frequent buffets because I know it's not beneficial. Oh I can, but I chose not to — and my hope is that you will review some things in your life, evaluate them and make your change today!

YES, YOU CAN!

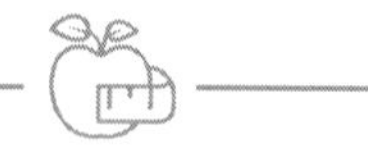

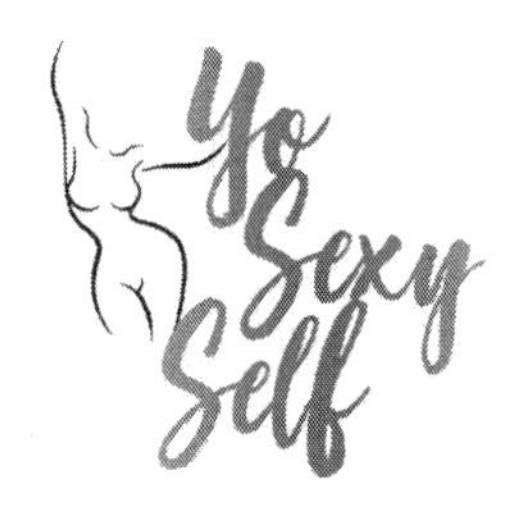

LET'S GET BUSY!

Section Two

NOURISH YOUR SEXY BODY

It's time to roll up your sleeves and get to work on that sexy body. In this section we will discuss the blueprint required for you to reshape your mind and your body. Let's take a look at the word "sexy." When you are sexy, you are sexually attractive to others. When your body is pleasing to the human eye, it causes others in the human species to linger and study you when they are observing it. They may use the following words to define you: seductive, desirable, alluring, sensual, sultry, provocative, tempting, or tantalizing.

While these are all nice adjectives, that's not the goal here. This sexiness I am discussing is one from within. A kind of confidence and assurance in yourself. Not a perverted – crass type. This is a good sexy. (smile)

Although that may make you feel good, the real benefit is you are healthier, feel good about yourself, and are better equipped to handle life's challenges. So let's get busy, getting you the body that you really want!

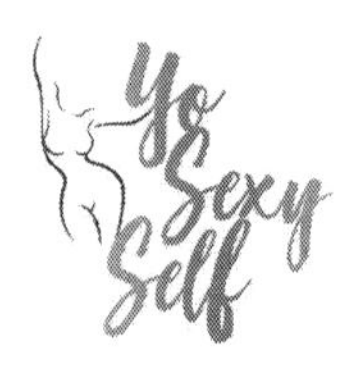

When you are sexy, you are sexually attractive to others.

Here are some key suggestions to get you moving in the right direction.

- **Change your relationship with food**
    - Food is fuel for your body
    - Journal your intake at the beginning to really see what / how much you are eating.
    - Don't use food for comfort
    - Get used to being satisfied not FULL
    - Let your food digest
    - Eat / Chew slowly

- **Meal planning**
    - Use a scale
    - Weigh your food to eliminate over/under eating
    - Meal planning helps with the temptation of visiting a fast food restaurant or grazing

- **Eating whole fresh food v. processed foods**
    - Eating whole foods help maintain your lifestyle. Its sustainable!
    - Cookie cutter diets aren't conducive for everyday life.

- Whole foods have a shorter shelf life than processed foods.
- Processed foods are full of preservatives and sodium.

MAIN NUTRIENTS

Protein

- Egg Whites
- Chicken Breast
- 99% Fat Free Turkey
- Turkey Cutlets
- White Fish-Cod, Tilapia,
- Salmon (good fats)
- Whey Isolate Protein
- Beans (Lentils, Black Beans)
- Edamame
- Tofu

Fats

- Avocado
- Flaxseed Oil
- Almonds
- Almond Butter
- Peanut Butter
- Coconut Oil

- Olive Oil
- Walnuts
- Cashews
- Sesame Oil

Carbs

- Oatmeal
- Brown Rice
- Quinoa
- Yams
- Red Potatoes
- Rice Cakes
- Cream of Wheat
- Honey

Fruit/Vegetables

- Blue / Black Berries
- Herbs / Peppers / Garlic / Shallots / Onions
- Green Beans
- Cucumbers
- Celery
- Spinach
- Asparagus
- Brussel Sprouts
- Broccoli

- Kale
- Zucchini
- Mustard and Collard Greens
- Romaine Lettuce
- Cabbage

Schedule the time to get meals prepped and workouts DONE! Possessing willpower is a must! THIS IS YOUR GOAL!

A CHANGE HAS TO COME

- **Mentally** – Your mental health is as important as your physical health. Maintain a proper balance and love YOU during your transformation.

- **Sleep** – Getting the proper amount of sleep should be a personal priority. Without it, your body can't perform at its highest level of proficiency.

- **Socially** – We are designed to be social creatures. With a few modifications to your eating habits you can continue to enjoy eating out, holidays with your family, and attending social events.

- **Nutrition** – Remember what you put in your body determines what you can get out of it. If you want optimum performance than you have to be selective about what kind of Fuel (food) goes into your body.

Now let's take a look at what you need to do initially to restructure your current eating habits and develop a healthier lifestyle.

YOUR EATING PLAN

- **Main Nutrients**
  - Proteins
  - Fruits and Vegetables
  - Fats
  - Carbohydrates
  - Herbs
  - Condiments and Other Miscellaneous Things We like to Eat and Drink
  - Developing a Personalized Meal Plan
- **Recipe Resources**

BACK TO WORK

As a busy professional with a family sometimes it may be hard for you to juggle everything. The answer is planning. Create a plan and stick to it! Here's a sample of how you can do all of the above and still work on your sexy body at the same time.

A Typical Work Day For A Working Mother

So you have to be in the office at 9 a.m. and you have two children to get to daycare first.

4:40 a.m. – wake up and get dressed

5:00 a.m. – one on one workout with your personal trainer

6:15 a.m. – back home shower, get the kids ready

Sample Meal Plan

6:15 a.m. – Post Workout Meal

- 1/3 cup of oatmeal or grits
- ¼ cup of blueberries or blackberries
- 3 egg whites and a whole egg

7:30 a.m. – out the door for drop off kids and to the office

9:30 a.m. - Breakfast

- *Cool Green Juice *Yo Sexy Self Juice Recipe*
- 3 cups of spinach
- 1 large green apple
- 4 celery stalks
- ½ in fresh turmeric root
- *135 calories

12:30 p.m. - Lunch

- *Bun Free Turkey Burger*

- 4oz of 99% fat free ground turkey breast
- Add veggies
- One heaping tablespoon of guacamole!
- Lay it on a leaf of lettuce

3:30 p.m. – Afternoon break

- Protein shake mixed with water and ice only!

6:30 p.m. - Dinner

- 1 cup cooked veggie stir fry
- 5 grilled jumbo shrimp or 5oz grilled fish

**about 1,300–1,500 calories*
**low calorie meals*

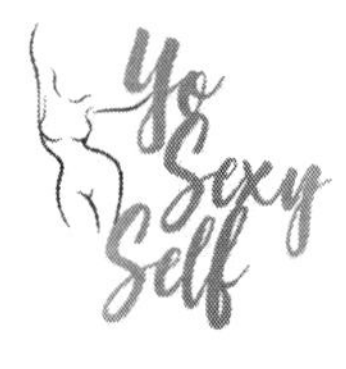

Create a plan and stick to it!

WATER IS A KEY FACTOR

H2O is of the utmost importance to your plan for healthy living. Your body is composed of approximately 60% water. It helps your body function and aids with digestion, kidney function, and skin elasticity.

Water aids with digestion it helps prevent constipation. Constipation is real and uncomfortable!

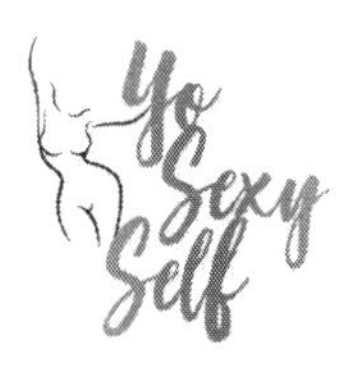

Water aids with digestion it helps prevent constipation.

Constipation is a condition in which there is difficulty in emptying the bowls usually associated with hardened feces.

WebMD says some of the causes of constipation are changes in your diet, not enough fiber or water intake, stress, overuse of laxatives, some medication and many others. I wanted to review some of the common ones.

Proper diet and exercise usually helps with constipation. It's a domino effect when you begin eating properly, like incorporating fiber and good fats in your diet, exercise will then help relieve stress and cause your blood to flow. When you follow The Sexy Body Blueprint you will be drinking lots of water and in doing all of this you should feel relief if you're experiencing constipation.

Kidney function can be impaired when your body is not getting enough water. Your urine concentration, color, and odor increases because the kidneys trap extra fluid for bodily functions. This can also cause kidney stones.

Skin is mostly water. Dehydration makes your skin look dry and wrinkled and can be improved with proper hydration

Water helps energize muscles if our cells don't maintain their balance of fluids and electrolytes shrivel, it can result in muscle fatigue, therefore; drink 1 gallon of water a day!

A supplement is something which completes or enhances something else when added to it. It can be in various forms such as multivitamins, powders, gels, etc. Check with your doctor, nutritionist, and/or trainer, wellness coach about what supplements could benefit you. The right supplements can help expedite your results. *Remember get professional advice and direction when adding supplements to your regime. Ask your physician!

- Most gyms will give you a one day or 3 day pass for free! Go online and check for offers before committing.
- Ask HR if there's a company allowance for gym memberships. Most large companies offer these perks in effort to motivate employees to stay healthy.
- Find out if there's actually a gym in your office building, where you can get a workout in before your work day starts or during lunch.
- Be Consistent – choose days you know you can commit to your program.

- Hire a certified - trainer / have a written-out plan
- Join a gym / CrossFit Box / Find a community center with a fitness center / Park with Bootcamps / Run Group / Dance Class / Zumba

GETTING STARTED!

- Wear Supportive Clothes
  - Sports Bras
  - Workout Tights
  - Headphones
  - Correct Shoes – sturdy, supports ankles, wide/narrow, runners get gait evaluation
- Gloves
- Back Belt
- Runners – Vaseline
- Gym Towel
- Yoga Mat
- ALWAYS TAKE H2O with you to a workout!

RECOVERY IS VERY IMPORTANT

Here are seven critical elements for recovery:

- Sleep!!!!
- Stretching / Foam Rolling

- Massage Therapy
- Chiropractor
- Ice Packs / Salonpas
- Have a COMPLETE rest day / Active Rest Day
- Eat AFTER workouts!

IN SUMMARY...

The Work Life Eat Balance Is:

- Get plenty of H2O
- Take the Necessary Supplements
- Start Training Your Body and Mind
- Recovering YOU is Critical to Your Ultimate Success in Life!

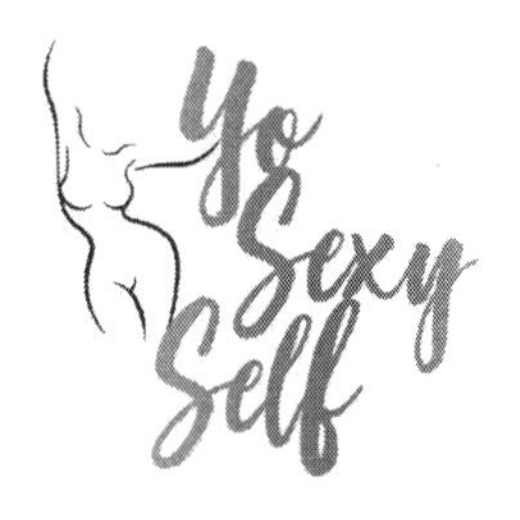

THE PLAN

I am so glad you have decided to go on this journey. There will be no more days going to the gym without a blueprint. To do anything successfully you must have a plan. This *Sexy Body Blueprint* will ensure you are getting a proper workout during each session.

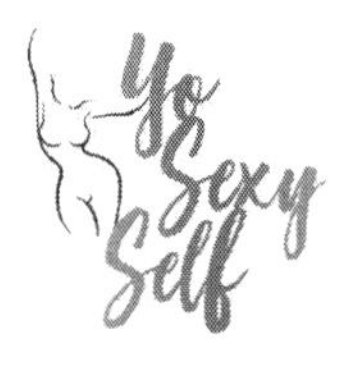

To do anything successfully you must have a plan.

You will exercise your entire body during the course of the week. This part of the blueprint will set the foundation for a new body. Here's a few reminders:

- Remember always make plans ladies!
- Plan your workout schedule.
- Plan what you are wearing to the gym!
- Create your meal plan or hire a professional to do this for you! Please don't skip this part.
- Schedule your bedtime! Your body needs the rest.

WHAT TO WEAR!

What you wear when you work out is so important. I have to admit, I want to look cute in the gym but not if it interferes with my workout. You must have on the right cute clothes AND SHOES.

- Bra
- Pants / Shorts

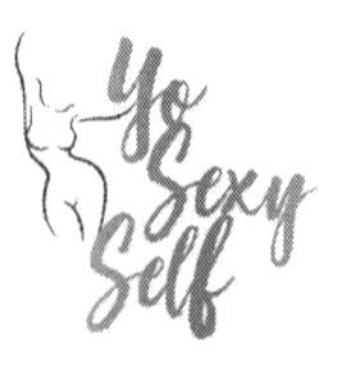

What you wear when you work out is so important.

- Good Shoes
- Gloves
- Cap

BRA

Having a good supportive bra is so essential. Sports bras are important to provide support and reduce movement. Lack of support and lots of downward movement can cause sagging – and we don't want sagging! A regular bra will not give you the same

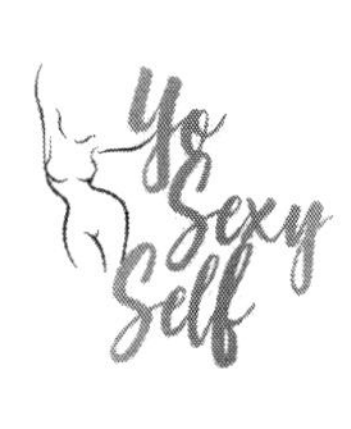

Sports bras are important to provide support and reduce movement.

support as a sport's bra. I see lots of ladies at the gym in regular T-Shirt bras. One time is okay, but don't make it a habit. Breast weight can range anywhere from ½ lb to 20 lbs, you really want to support your breast.

For Example: If you're working out and you don't have proper support, your breasts are pulling you forward. Your form will be compromised altering your posture. GET A SPORTS BRA!

Find a bra made with nice mesh and wicking breathable material. This type of material will draw moisture away from your body. Look for CoolMax try to stay away from all cotton.

PANTS/SHORTS

You must have some cute well supporting workout pants! Cute is subjective but supportive, AIN'T. Supportive in that they are thick enough to hold your body. Your pants or workout tights should be made with a nice material that will keep you modest. I have seen black tights that are so thin you can see a lady's white underwear.

If you are jumping rope or performing a jump squat you want tights that will compress, hold, and support your body. Not have you jiggling and shaking.

Remember wear breathable fabrics. Gray materials are cute but know ALL YOUR sweat stains will be very visible. If you're like me and you sweat in your crevices, you may want to consider wearing dark colors or busy prints which won't draw attention DIRECTLY to your lady parts. Okay moving on…

Shorts are my favorite bottoms to work out in because I have extremely long legs and feel freer when I move. They can be awesome for leg day so you can see your progress when you train. I love to run in shorts even in the winter because they keep me cool and I don't tire so quickly.

Tights or shorts it doesn't matter wear what makes you feel SEXY!

SHOES

Good shoes are most important. Your feet are like your body's foundation. They balance your body's weight, help your posture, and help you get from one place to another. Your feet are so important you must protect and provide them with adequate support!

Workout shoes should be comfortable, functional, and serve the purpose.

When performing an exercise your ankles should be supported.

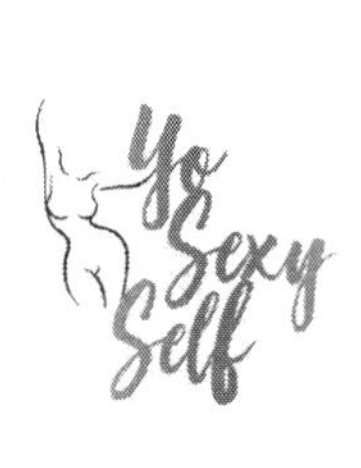

> Your feet are like your body's foundation. They balance your body's weight, help your posture, and help you get from one place to another.

Aerobic or Running shoes should have thick cushioned soles to absorb some of the shock of your workout with a good supportive heel so your gait is not compromised. These shoes should also be made of breathable fabric.

When it comes to lifting I like a flat sole shoe that will help keep my feet in one place. While doing squats, deadlifting, or standing and doing shoulder presses, you want your feet stationary!

GLOVES

Gloves are an optional part of your workout but they do have their advantages especially in a gym setting. They give you a better grip when your hands become sweaty. They also can be more comfortable than going barehanded and some of them offer wrist support during weightlifting. During inclement weather, you may want to use them to keep your hands warm when you are working out outside or running.

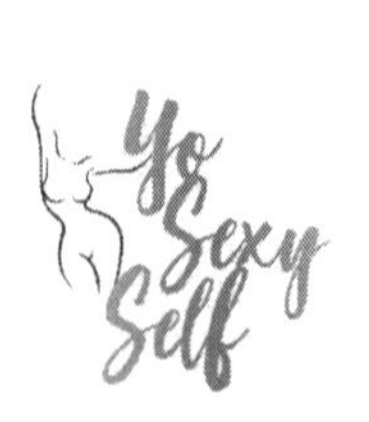

They give you a better grip when your hands become sweaty.

CAP

A cap is also optional, but it can come in handy when you are working out or running in inclement weather. Also, if your hair is long and has a tendency to get caught in things, you may want to wear a cap around the gym to avoid your hair being caught in the equipment.

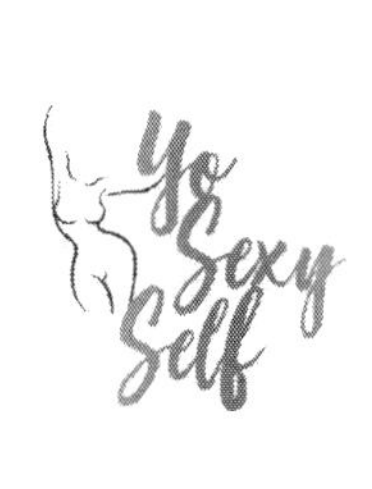

A cap is also optional, but it can come in handy when you are working out or running in inclement weather.

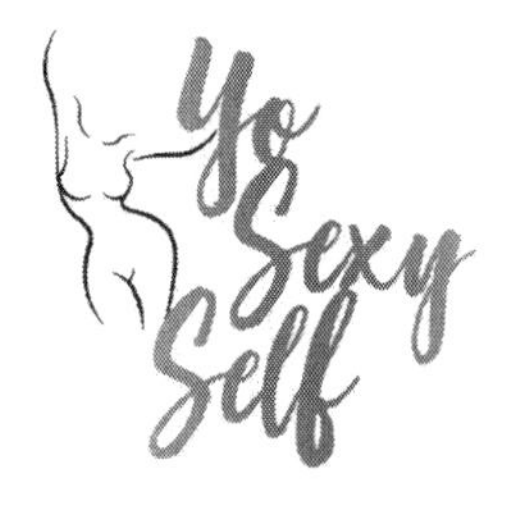

THE SEXY BODY BLUEPRINT

Let's get physical, physical
I want to get physical
Let's get into physical
Let me hear your body talk, your body talk
Let me hear your body talk[2]

"Physical" is song sung by British-born Australian singer Olivia Newton-John. It was released in September 1981 and spent 10 weeks at number one on the Billboard Hot 100. I would like to invite you to make it your personal theme song when you start on your journey to a sexy body.

Let's get you physical with a sample workout schedule!

SAMPLE WORKOUT SCHEDULE

- Mondays – Legs
- Tuesdays – Arms
- Wednesdays – Abs / Back

2. *Olivia Newton-Johns Greatest Hits* [CD]. (1982). MCA Records.

- Thursdays – Legs / Cardio
- Friday – Conditioning
- Saturday – Active Rest
- Sunday – Rest

MONDAY - LEGS

(Glutes/Hamstrings)

We work glutes and hamstrings on Mondays because Sunday is our day of rest and most of the time if there is a slip up on the meal plan, it happened over the weekend. Your glutes are the largest muscles in your body. They consist of the gluteus maximus, gluteus, medius, and gluteus minimus. The maximus is what shapes your booty! Working these muscles will burn a lot of calories while causing the least amount of damage control. Hamstrings are the 3 muscles behind the thigh. They are the semitendinosus, semimembranosus, and the biceps femoris.

When I am training someone and they have a bad back or poor posture – this is a muscle group I really focus on because your glutes and hamstrings support your lower back. If you get those stronger – trust me it will help with those issues. It will take patience and consistency.

Sample Glute/Hamstring Workout

- 12 - X 3 Body Weight Squat
- 15 - 20 X 3 Hip Thrust

- 12 - 15 X 3 Step Ups
- 12 - 15 X 3 Clamshells
- 12 - 15 X 3 Standing Kickbacks
- 30 sec X 3 Jump Squats

TUESDAYS - ARMS

(Shoulders/Biceps/Triceps)

Toned arms are so sexy on a lady! I think of Michelle Obama or Angela Bassett when I think of nice toned arms. So Tuesday is the day we dedicate to getting our arms tight and right. The shoulders are the place we carry most of our stress. In the fitness world, we call shoulders – delts. The deltoid muscles consist of an anterior (front) head, middle (lateral) head, and rear (posterior) head. It's important to always stretch before any workout but especially stretch your shoulders. The increased flexibility in your shoulders will increase your strength and decrease the amount of load that your bones, ligaments, and joints have to bear. Biceps are those muscles below the delts. It's important to give these babies some attention too. Although these are the muscles men typically OVERWORK. Triceps (muscles) have lateral, long, and medial heads. Now this is probably one of my least favorite muscles to train but it's so important not to miss this one. Fat tends to accumulate RIGHT HERE on us ladies. That's why we must work these muscles. To annihilate the fats!

Sample Shoulder / Biceps / Triceps Workout

- 12 - 15 X 3 Seated Overhead Press
- 12 - 15 X 3 Cable Upright Row
- 12 - 15 X 3 Front Raises
- 12 - 15 X 3 Barbell Curls
- 12 - 15 X 3 Alternating Hammer Curls
- 12 - 15 X 3 Dumbbell Kickbacks
- 12 - 15 X 3 Cable Kickbacks
- 12 - 15 X 3 Machine Dips

WEDNESDAY - ABS / BACK

(Abdominals Core / Back)

The workouts are not too sexy but your back will be once you commit to these exercises. These exercises will help get rid of those "love handles" and the back fat we really don't want to follow us. The major muscles in your back are the latissimus dorsi (lat), teres major, rhomboids, and the deep erectors.

Abs – Core! I have learned to love to work my abs. Let me tell you why–my core became my foundation. The stronger it got the stronger I became! It helps with balance, posture, and form. It doesn't take a lot and it doesn't take long but it does take consistency.

Your abdominal muscles include rectus abdominis, external obliques, internal obliques, and transverse abdominis.

It is crucial you dedicate time and patience on this workout. Breathe! Most people hold their breath when working abs – DON'T DO IT. You could pass out. Inhale and exhale as you move. Allow the oxygen to get into your body.

Sample Ab (Core)/Back Workout

- 15 - 20 X 3 Crunch
- 15 - 20 X 3 Laying Heel Touches
- 15 - 20 X 3 Crossover Crunch
- 12 - 15 Lat Pulldown
- 12 - 15 Bent – over Row
- 30 - 40 sec X 3 Superman Hold
- 30 - 40 sec Plank

THURSDAY – LEGS/CARDIO

(Quadriceps)

Quadriceps, or thighs! Thighs are made up of the vastus lateralis, vastus medialis, vastus intermedius, and rectus femoris.

There are benefits to training quads, it promotes stability in the knee and you burn a lot of calories! Who doesn't like a pair of pretty toned thighs in a pair of shorts!

Day two of training legs ladies, we typically hold most of our adipose tissue (fat) in our lower extremities. So I always train myself and my clients' legs twice a week. Thursdays are not as strenuous as Monday because I mix in cardio!

Sample Quad/Cardio Workout

15 -20 Leg Press

30 - 40 sec Toe Taps

10 - 15 Walking Lunges

30 - 40 sec Squat Jacks

12 -15 Leg Extensions

30 -40 sec Jumping Jacks

FRIDAY - CONDITIONING

When I think of a lady with excellent body conditioning I picture Angelina Jolie in Lara Croft Tomb Raider or Danai Gurira "Okoye" in Black Panther. These ladies are agile, strong, and sexy! Their bodies are in condition. It takes a unique mix of strength, cardio, and core training to perform the stunts in those movies.

I make sure to dedicate a session in my training schedule to this type of training. It can be intense but the payoff is awesome – you will also see the benefits in your other workouts.

Sample Conditioning Workout

- 30 sec X 4 Jumping Jacks
- 30 sec X 4 Toe Taps
- 30 sec X 4 Bear Crawls

- 30 sec X 4 Battle Ropes
- 30 sec X 4 Medicine Ball Slam

SATURDAY - ACTIVE REST

Okay you have worked super hard for 5 straight days your body needs to kind of settle down – BUT NOT COMPLETELY.

During an active rest day your body can start to really recover from all the workouts from the week. Take this day to move but with the same intensity as a regular workout day.

Active rest suggestions:

- Walking (walking the dog)
- Bike ride
- Yoga
- Swim – excellent!
- Go for a hike
- Gardening

SUNDAY - REST!

Having rest days doesn't mean sitting on the couch munching. This day is for meal preparation and taking time to recharge your batteries.

Resting is just as important as the workouts themselves. Your muscles, nerves, bones, and connective tissues need time to recover and get STRONGER.

Rest can help prevent injury because your body is being overused. You compromise your immune system when you don't rest. Your immune system is constantly activating to repair muscles and joints. Without the rest your immune system can't keep up and you run the risk of injury.

Most people don't have a problem with taking a rest day though!

Now it's time to work on your eating. I have included a sample meal schedule below that will guarantee you will have the fuel needed to get "physical."

SAMPLE MEAL SCHEDULE

TIME	ACTIVITY
4:40 am	Pre-Workout
5:00 am	One-on-One Workout with Personal Trainer
6:15 am	Meal One
9:30 am	Meal Two
12:30 pm	Meal Three
3:30 pm	Meal Four
6:30 pm	Meal Five

Tips to Consider:

- **Have your meals prepared.**
    - IF you're not prepared you will eat anything.
    - Hunger hurts and you lose all rationality.

- **Don't Graze!**
  - Grazing is defined as eating small amounts of foods continuously.
  - Grazing is a terrible habit – which is difficult to break.
  - When you graze you don't eat a full meal you are eating mindlessly.
  - You can become malnourished- because most of the time you are not eating a balanced meal and providing your body with the proper nutrition it needs.
  - You can be overweight and malnourished.

- **Don't eat out –** eat the food you prepared. You know what's inside your food. You can ask the restaurant not to add certain things, but you ultimately have no control over how something is prepared.
  - This is crucial for the beginning of your journey so you can get acclimated to eating a new way
  - Prepare your own foods – this is a lifestyle change REMEMBER!

- **Don't skip meals –** keep your metabolism going by consuming healthy meals.

- **Drink plenty of water**

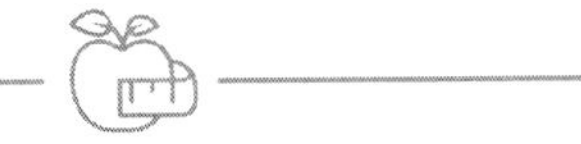

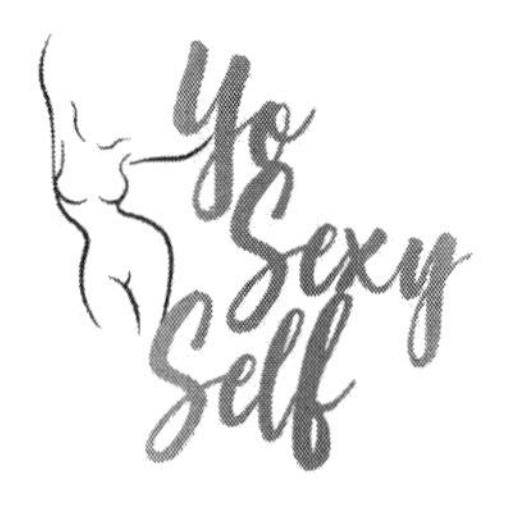

LOOKING IN THE MIRROR

When I started my journey several years ago, I never imagined I would someday help others achieve their goals to develop a sexy body. Now I have a business and I've officially written my first book, *The Sexy Body Blueprint*. Everything I've done has required a lot of self-discipline, faith, and perseverance. I wish I could tell you it was easy but it wasn't, it required a tremendous amount of sacrifice. Now, as I look in the mirror, it was all worth it.

You're worth it! If it means I helped you as a result of my journey, then it was truly worth my efforts. I value your right to live an abundant life and the highest good I can do here on earth is help you be the healthiest and sexiest individual possible.

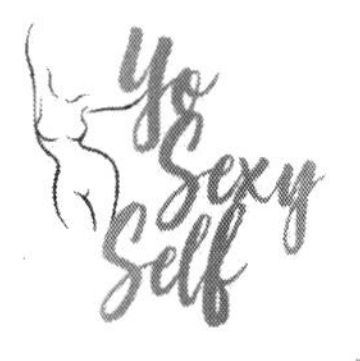

You're worth it!

I believe you can do anything you set your mind to do. I did and you possess the very same "can do" power. Don't waste the time and money you've invested in this book. Use it to become the best and sexiest YOU ever!

Patrina

TESTIMONIALS

Teoka S's Testimonial

"I am honored and overjoyed to recommend Patrina. She is a premier trainer, mentor, and friend. Her technique is truly holistic and she will mold your mind, BODY, and spirit. She is a warrior and she will help you conquer your fears, negative ego and unhealthy habits both physically and spiritually. I will use her title to describe her attributes that makes her the best trainer ever.....

– Everything that follows this line is absolutely facts!

B – Brilliant, Beast at Body re-imaging

E – Energetic and Encouraging

S – Spirit-filled and Spectacular

E – Excellent and Extraordinary

X – Xtravagant and X-ray vision

Y – Youthful and truly YOURS

The return on investment with Patrina is matchless."

Ashley G's Testimonial

"It was 14 months after I gave birth to my son when I started working out with Patrina and, let me just say it was God's intervention connecting us. Up to that point I had worked out in the gym and done boot camps but I wasn't eating right and not working out properly. It frustrated me and knew I needed help from someone but I didn't know where to start or who to trust. Patrina was working out at our neighborhood gym and I remember thinking, wow that is discipline. Wonder if she trains people? To my surprise few weeks later, she started a boot camp. I went to every boot camp she offered and finally asked for help. She listened to what my goals were which was to get back to my pre-baby weight and designed a plan that worked for me and my lifestyle. With her help, I learned to work out properly, what to eat, how much, and most importantly I gained a friend. Patrina is patient, holds you accountable and simply the best at what she does. Oh, and I got to the goal and still implement her nutrition and workout plans."

Shayla O's Testimonial

"Patrina is hands down the best fitness coach I have ever worked with! She not only educated me on health and fitness but also was a great source of support and fellowship for me during my transition to becoming healthy and fit. I love how Patrina understands how to work with female clients like myself. With her workouts you get fast results without injury which keeps you motivated to reach your goals. I saw dramatic results in just 6 weeks; I saw definition, became stronger, and had more endurance. In her book, The Sexy Body Blueprint, she provides guidance and knowledge to help you reach your fitness and health goals. It's a must-read for anyone who wants to improve their fitness!"

Leslie D's Testimonial

"It is a privilege and a blessing to train with Patrina. Besides her infinite knowledge, she has a wonderfully calming and spiritual energy that will motivate you. She is a true gift!"

Crystal L's Testimonial

"Patrina Mosca is a gift that keeps on giving. She is committed to showing people you can become a better version of yourself and love it. Her attention to detail is incredible and she always keeps in mind what's best for you as an individual. The day I started to work with her I was in between wanting to give up at the same time. My weight was 183 lbs. She met me where I was and challenged me with compassion to do the work and gave me her word if I put my best foot forward, it will work for me. Although some exercises may be difficult, she shows you how she wants it done and make sure you do it with great form. One of the things I love is if something is too difficult she quickly thinks of a way to change the exercise to fit you and still get the same results. I thought I was just getting a trainer but I received much more. She has taught me discipline, pushed me to become better, and held me accountable even in my weakest times. She has taught me no matter

Crystal L's Testimonial (cont.)

what goes on in life you can't give up on you. Patrina has shown me everything works together, the way you eat, what you eat, how you exercise, the rest you receive and your mindset. What I admire about her the most is she doesn't teach you to do as she said but she leads by example and that above everything else pushes me to work harder. I now weigh about 153 lb. and I'm still working. Thank You Big Sister Be Sexy!"

Andria M's Testimonial

"I hired Patrina as a trainer knowing I had the potential to be better, but not exactly understanding how to DO better. I bought the will and desire, but Patrina supplied important tools that were missing - strength/interval/circuit training as well as focus, accountability, and consistency. She met me at the level of fitness I had and helped me to gain strength and endurance at an appropriate pace always challenging me to compete with myself by consistently raising my own bar. She also taught me how the body's optimal state can be achieved through a combination of nutrition and exercise. The best thing about Patrina is she cares about her clients as people - this is clearly evident in what she does, and how she does it."

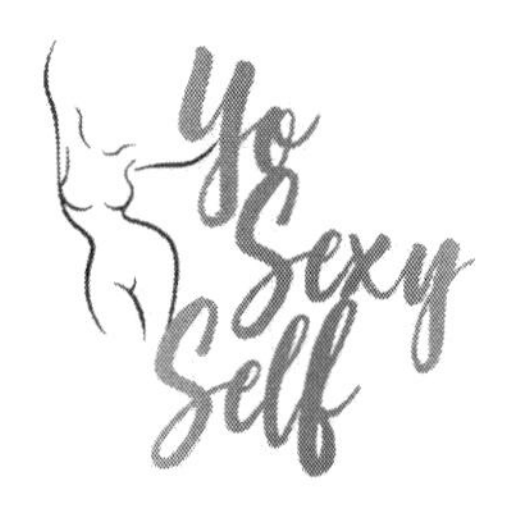

ABOUT the AUTHOR

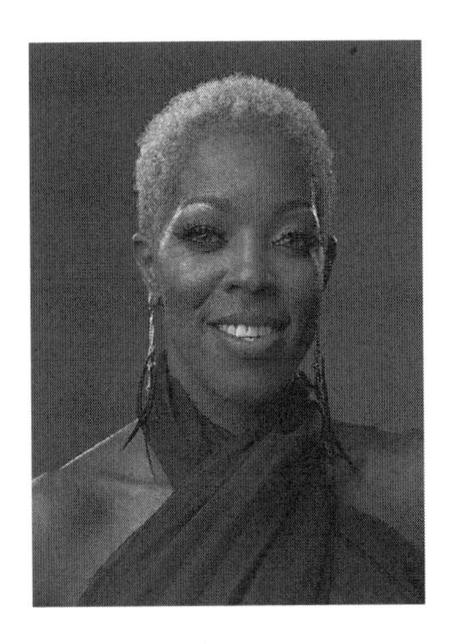

PATRINA MOSCA is a wife, mother, lover of people and all things fitness. Her son Jaylin, the oldest, and daughters Mia, Jamila, Laura, and Allegra, are her greatest contributions to this world. She is a native Houstonian and member of the Lighthouse Church under the leadership of Pastor Keion Henderson and First Lady Felicia Henderson. She loves her church family! She also loves serving the elderly and those in need.

Her husband, Fausto and Patrina met in Houston. Running brought them together and it's something that they still enjoy doing together. They train, meal prep, and run races together. Fausto is Italian, the couple enjoy blending their cultures and traditions. It's what makes their relationship so fun and unique.

Patrina is an avid runner, but her favorite workouts take place in the weight rooms! She loves to lift. Her body responds well to weight-lifting. It's the foundation of her company's training methods. She is a figure competitor. She has placed and won in the NSL and Musclemannia natural leagues. Patrina enjoys the competition process and the overall experience. She is also a certified fitness trainer, nutritionist, and licensed massage therapist.

In 2019, Patrina is adding the moniker "author," to her list of accomplishments. She will be releasing her first book, *The Sexy Body Blueprint* in February of this year.